Yoga Breath Practices

Yoga Tools for Kids:

Creating Healthy Minds & Bodies

Series

❖ *Yoga Breath Practices*

❖ *Mindfulness & Meditation for Children*

❖ *Yoga Games & Activities Volume 1*

❖ *Yoga Games & Activities Volume 2*

❖ *Yoga Lesson Plans for Kids*

❖ *Yoga by the Month*

❖ *Mantra Affirmation Cards*

Yoga Breath Practices:

Teaching Kids the Importance of Breath

Yoga Breath Practices:
Teaching Kids the Importance of Breath

FIRST EDITION

Yoga Tools for Kids:
Creating Healthy Minds & Bodies

Series – BOOK 1

Soft Cover ISBN: 979-8-9887936-1-8

Dedicated to Our Children

the ones we taught,

have yet to meet,

and the ones we raised.

OMtastic Yoga

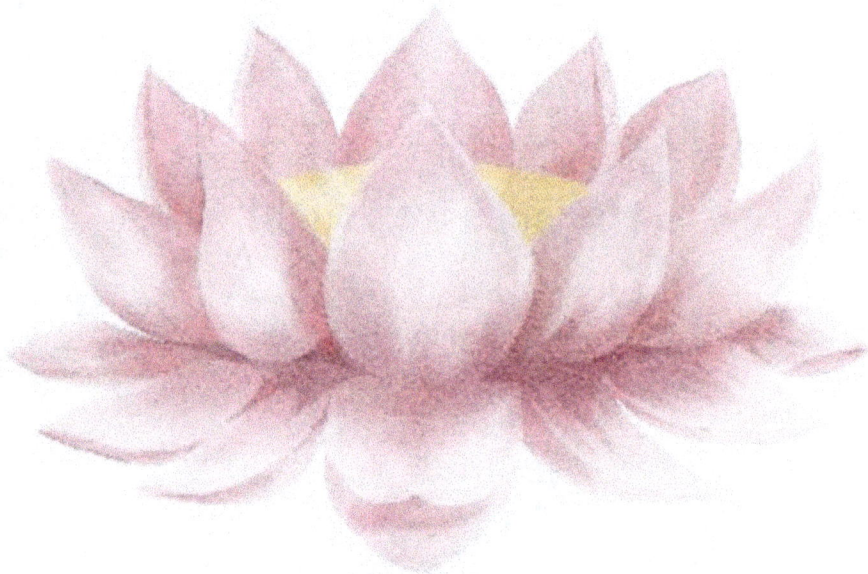

Make each day your

masterpiece!

John Wooden

TABLE OF CONTENTS

Just Breathe!

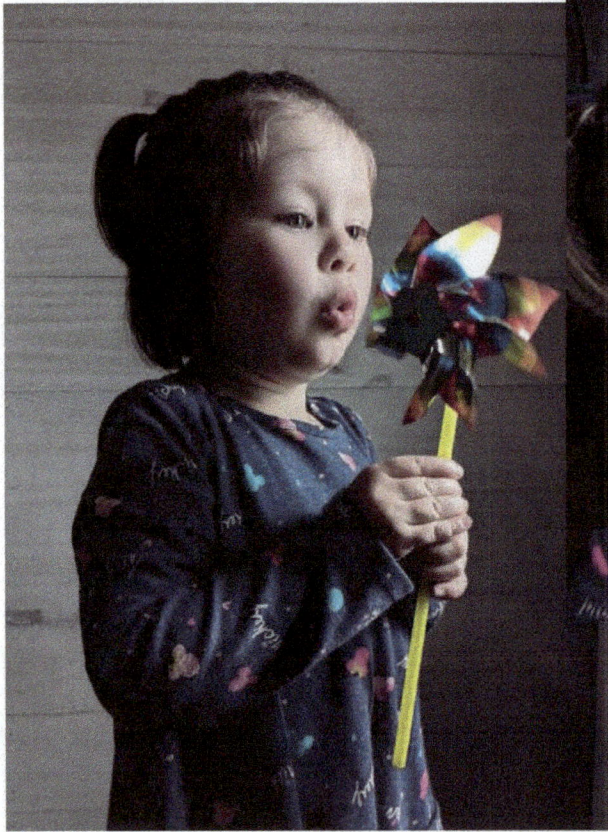

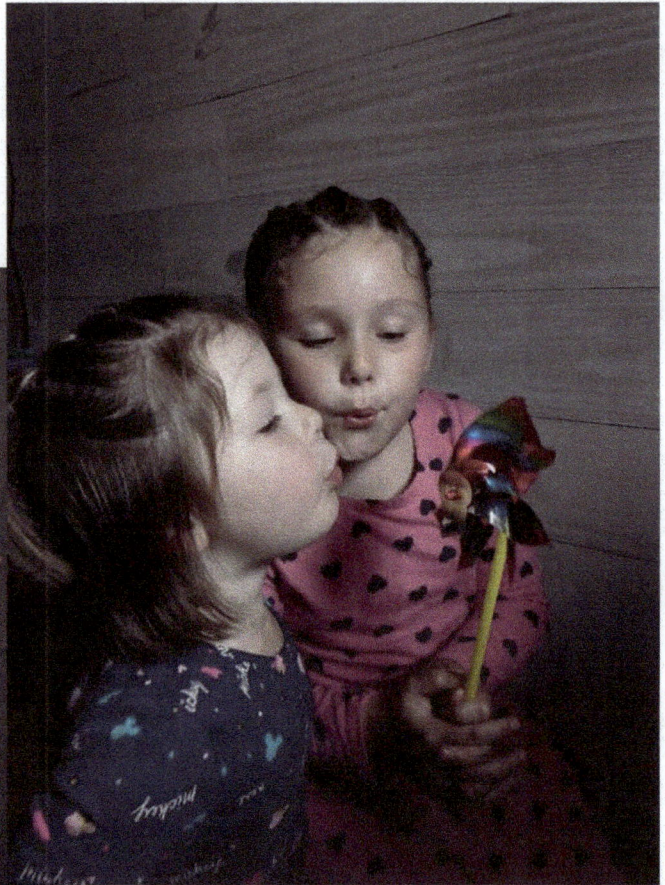

Photos courtesy of Janice Pratt

Introduction

Namasté.

Welcome to Yoga Breath Practices.

The breath is an important part of the autonomic nervous system. We breathe every minute of every day and don't even think about it. We breathe in our sleep. We breathe when we are exercising. We breathe throughout the day. Everyone does it. All the time.

However, we can also voluntarily control our breath. We can hold our breath. We can speed up the breath and we can slow it down. This is a powerful superpower and it has a powerful benefit to the body.

When we introduce this superpower to kids, we start with practices that draw attention to the movement of the breath and practices that help kids to notice how they feel when the normal pattern of the breath changes.

As children get older, we talk about the effect that changes in the breath have on the body and our emotions. For example, when we are afraid, the breath might be faster and shorter. When we are relaxed, it might be longer and slower.

Finally, we teach the effect of the breath on the nervous system. When the breath is slower and deeper, this is a sign to the nervous system that we are safe. This is the place we want to learn to be as often as we can!

With children, play is part of learning. In this bundle of breath practices, there are many different ways to bring attention to the breath, but one key to each practice is the element of exploration and fun.

My hope with these practices, is to provide lifelong tools that help children be more regulated in their nervous systems, and help them learn to make choices and decisions from this place of calm.

With gratitude,

Janice Pratt

We welcome your feedback!
play@omtastic-yoga.com
www.omtastic-yoga.com

Follow Omtastic Yoga on Facebook
for events and lots of free ideas!

Principles of Yoga

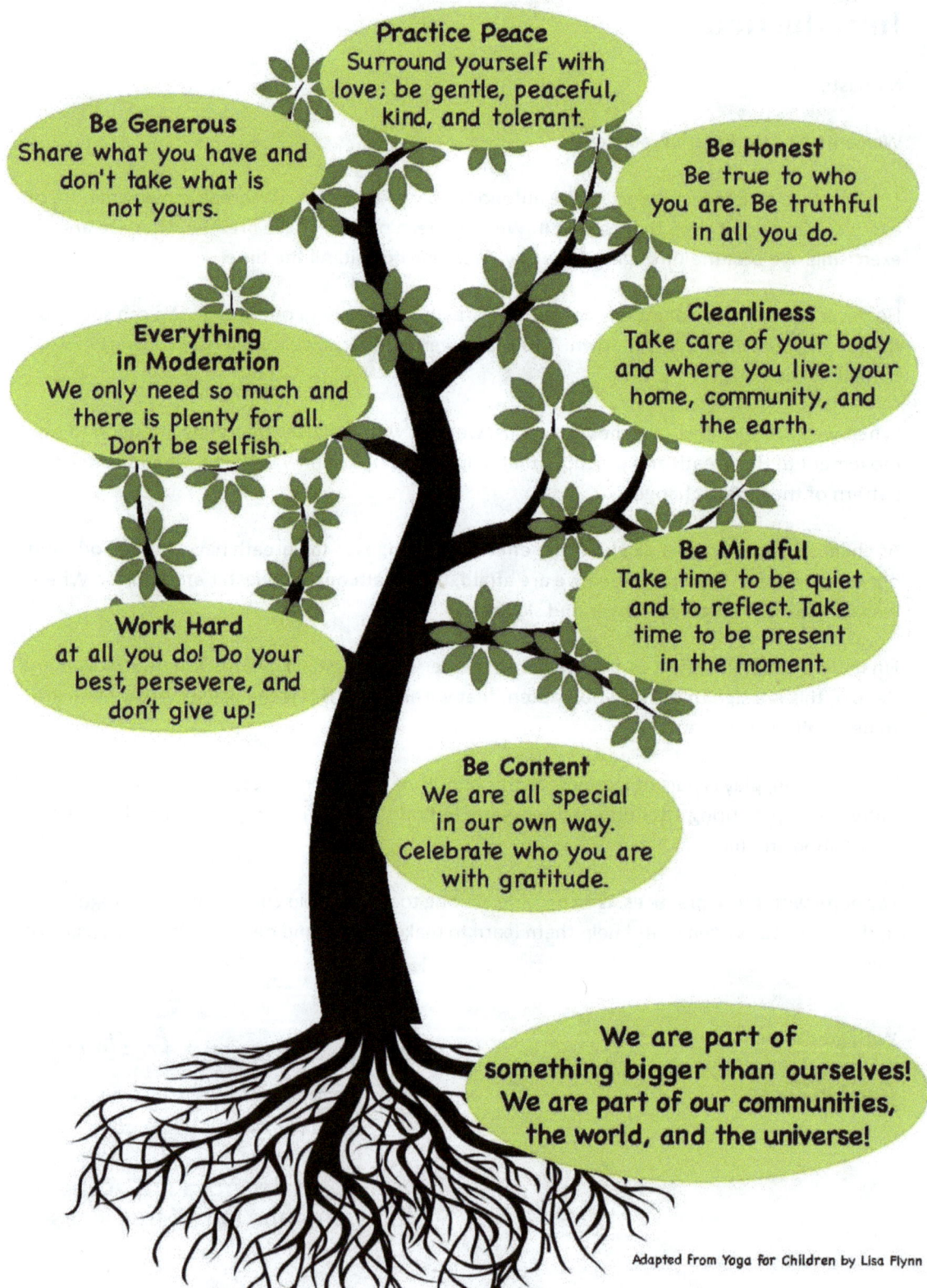

Practice Peace
Surround yourself with love; be gentle, peaceful, kind, and tolerant.

Be Generous
Share what you have and don't take what is not yours.

Be Honest
Be true to who you are. Be truthful in all you do.

Everything in Moderation
We only need so much and there is plenty for all. Don't be selfish.

Cleanliness
Take care of your body and where you live: your home, community, and the earth.

Be Mindful
Take time to be quiet and to reflect. Take time to be present in the moment.

Work Hard
at all you do! Do your best, persevere, and don't give up!

Be Content
We are all special in our own way. Celebrate who you are with gratitude.

We are part of something bigger than ourselves! We are part of our communities, the world, and the universe!

Adapted from Yoga for Children by Lisa Flynn

Yoga Class and Our Agreements

In order to have fun in yoga, we need to agree on acceptable behavior in class.

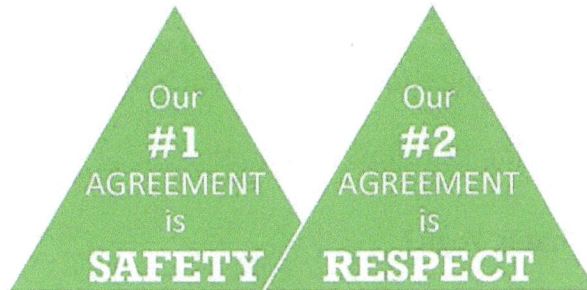

SAFETY
We try new poses together, with supervision.
We keep hands to ourselves.
We stay on our mats unless told otherwise.

RESPECT
RESPECT for OURSELVES
RESPECT for OTHERS
RESPECT for our ENVIRONMENT

This is a good time to go over other housekeeping items. Don't make the list too long. Generally, we have 2 things that should be done at the beginning or before class:

- Use the restroom
- Fill your water bottle

You can structure a routine that covers what to do when entering the yoga room (where to put their backpacks if they are coming from school, where to put their shoes, designate a place to eat their snack, etc.)

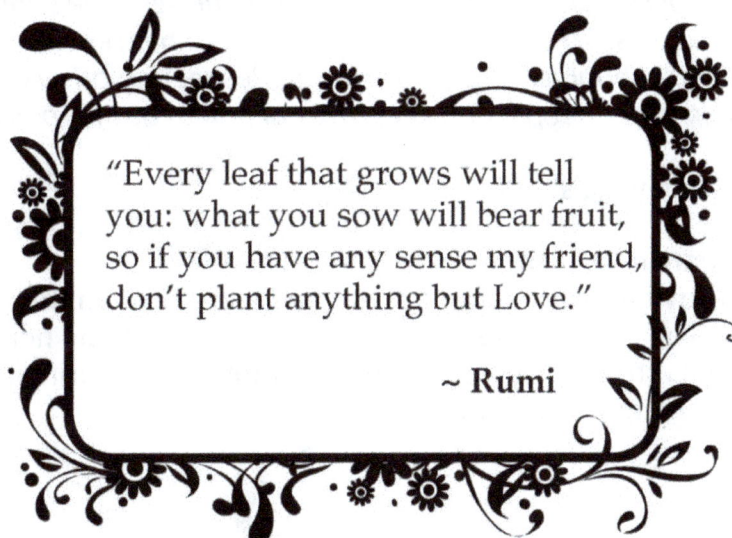

"Every leaf that grows will tell you: what you sow will bear fruit, so if you have any sense my friend, don't plant anything but Love."

~ Rumi

Your First Yoga Class

When beginning a new series such as "Planting Seeds" or any other curriculum, you will probably want to begin with a brief introduction of "What is Yoga?" If this is your first class with a new group of students, you will want to introduce yourself to the class and facilitate introducing themselves to each other, as well.

You may lead your own discussion or follow this one:

Opening Discussion: What is Yoga?

The word "yoga" means "union."

Question: What are we bringing together in yoga?

Possible Answers: *Breath and movement, mind and body, friends*

What we learn in yoga, we can take with us as we move throughout our day. We can use our breath to calm ourselves, we can use poses to make our bodies work well and feel good, and, most importantly, we can treat everyone like they have a special "light" inside of them, which we see and respect.

Question: Why do we practice yoga?

Possible Answers: *To help our bodies and minds relax, to calm ourselves, to be physically healthy, etc.* **Yoga is good for our brains and our bodies.**

Question: How can practicing yoga make the world a better place?

Possible Answers: *When we are feeling and doing our best, we share that energy with those around us. Treating others as we wish to be treated will make our friends and family feel happier and appreciated. Respecting others and our surroundings will help other people and keep the earth a beautiful place to live.*

Question: Where did yoga start?

Answer: Yoga began in India thousands of years ago.
Yogis began to study the world around them and learn how animals and nature worked together. They learned ways to move their bodies to be healthy, and how to make their brains strong by being **mindful**. Mindfulness is bringing concentration and focus to one thing at a time.

OM tastic Yoga

CHAPTER 1

BREATH PRACTICES FOR PRESCHOOLERS

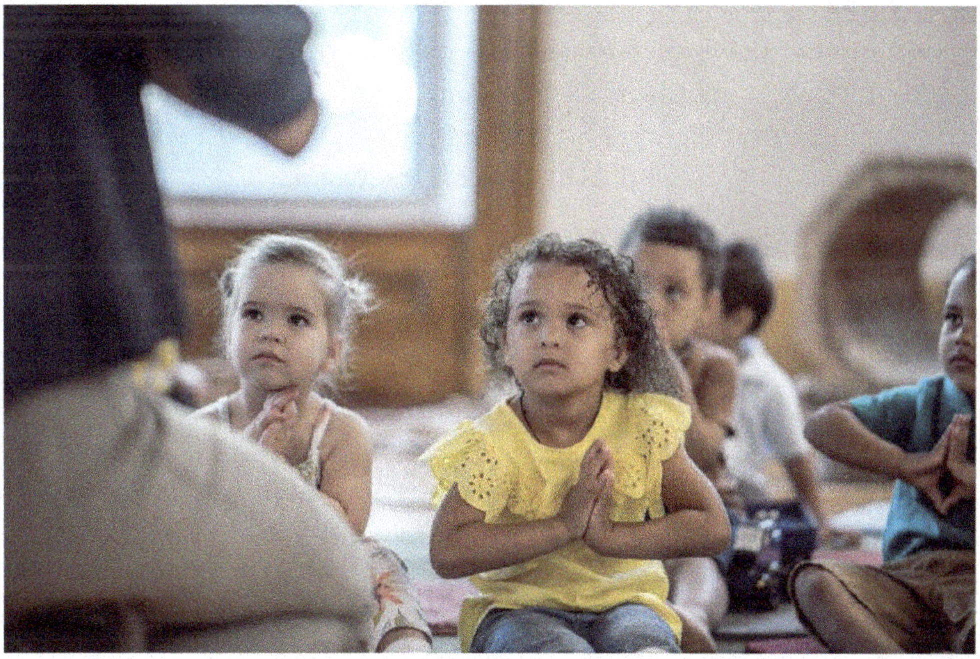

Image courtesy of Canva, Public Domain

OMtastic Yoga

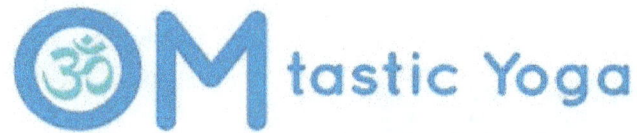

Breath Practices for Preschoolers

Blowing Bubbles

Bubble are great fun for all ages. For young children who are just exploring their breath, bubbles can be a little challenging.

One aspect that makes this easier is to have a quality bubble solution. I like to make my own using Dawn dish washing solution and a bit of glycerin. This makes the bubbles a bit more elastic and long lasting and they don't seem to pop as quickly on the wand.

Also with this age, it is nice that everyone has their own bubble wand. If parents are available, they can hold the bubble solution so there are fewer spills. However, be prepared for spills!

Have clean up supplies handy or go outside if it is available.

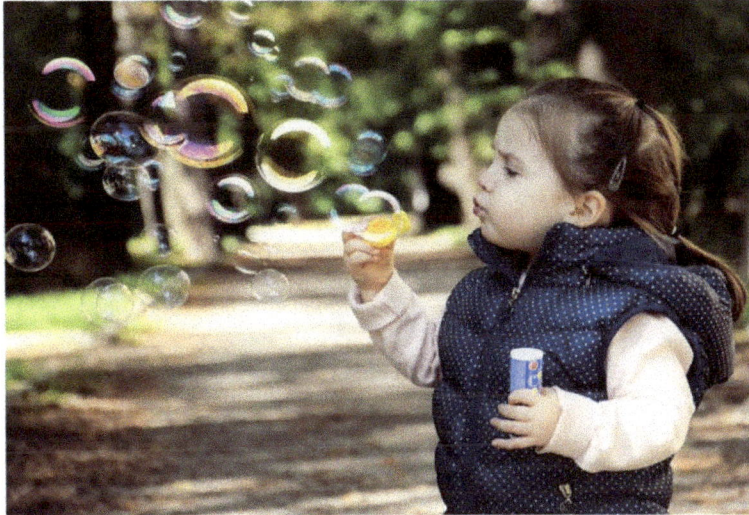

Image courtesy of Canva, Public Domain

Options for Bubble Blowing

- Everyone has their own wand and bubble solution.
- After they are blowing bubbles confidently, they can try to catch bubbles on their wands.
- You can find giant wands and children wave the wands.
- Parents blow bubbles and the children chase the bubbles.
- Place the bubble solution in a dish and have children blow through a straw to make bubbles in the dish.
- Make up a bubble game.

Websites for Bubble Solutions:

Artful Parent
https://artfulparent.com/

Happy Hooligans
https://happyhooligans.ca/

☉M tastic Yoga

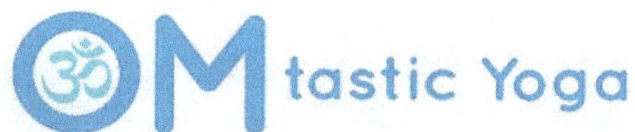

Breath Practices for Preschoolers

~

Breathing Buddies

~

I like using a script with this breath, especially if you have never used Breathing Buddies. Of course, once you are comfortable with the routine, you can be creative with it and give it your own spin.

With young kids, it is great to build up the excitement with the idea that the stuffies are special friends that pick a special student each time they come out. This is fun to do with kids all the way through elementary school. I have even done a version with older kids where you place an eye pillow or bean bag on their stomach.

The idea is that they can learn to breathe into the lower part of their lungs and really sense into where they can feel their breath in their body.

You will need small beanie babies or stuffies for this activity.

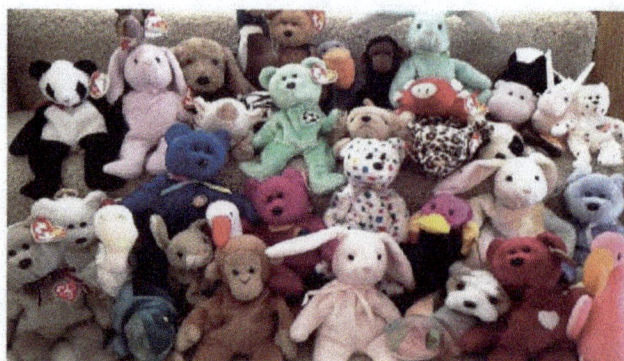

Image courtesy of Canva, Public Domain

Script

Begin by lying down on your back. Close your eyes or look softly at the ceiling.
Let your hands rest beside you.

Today, we have some special friends visiting us. They are very shy and, if you wiggle
or talk, they often run and hide and won't come back out.
So let's be super quiet.

When they hear that it is very quiet, they make their way out of my special basket and
land right on your belly.

Now, each time they come to visit, these special friends somehow know who they want
to spend time with. So each time they visit, you might get to meet a new friend.

It is really exciting if you can keep your eyes closed the whole time and
meet your friend at the end of this relaxation.

Now, as I walk around and place a special friend on your belly, just notice
how the weight of your friend feels.

Ever so gently, see if you can bring your breath deep into your belly so that your belly
rises, giving your friend a gentle ride up and a gentle ride down as you exhale.

Do this a few more times, lifting your friend up with your inhale and down
with your exhale.

Now, very slowly reach your arms over your head and point your toes and take a long
stretch.

Hug your knees into your chest and wrap your arms around your
knees, hugging your friend in tight so they feel very safe.

Take 2 or 3 "rock and rolls" on your spine, coming to "criss cross applesauce."
Meet your new friend.

Remember if you get loud, your friend might get sacred and run away,
so keep your voice very soft or off.

Bring your Beanie Baby's hands or fins or wings together in namaste hands.

Namaste.

OMtastic Yoga

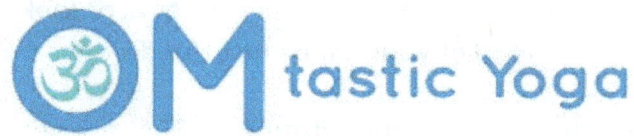

Breath Practices for Preschoolers

Candle Breath

This activity can be done with students when you notice a particularly high level of energy in your group, or when there is a great deal of conflict.

Some great times might be:

- before you move to a quiet activity when children are very loud
- after students have gone through a transition
- when you need to get attention after a high energy activity

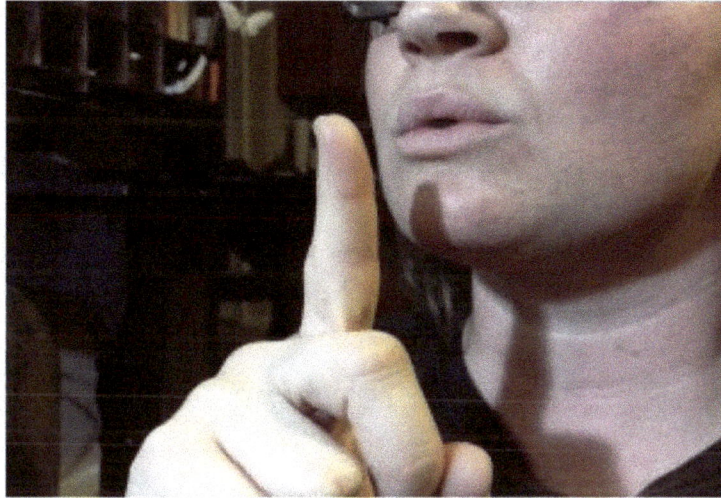

Image courtesy of Canva, Public Domain

Script for Candle Breath

Have students sit in a circle on a rug or, if space is limited, they can stand in a circle.

Turn off or dim overhead lights, if possible.

Take your hands and interlace your fingers. Hold up just the pointer fingers to make them look like a candle. For very young kids, you can use just one hand and hold up the pointer finger.

Ask everyone to take a breath in with you, and blow it out very slowly through pursed lips, like you are blowing on a candle. You can repeat several times until you notice the energy of the group changing.

You can change up the breath by having kids blow soft or hard, slow or fast.

End the activity with the soft, slow out-breath for the last couple of breaths.

OMtastic Yoga

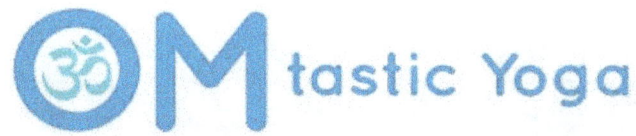

Breath Practices for Preschoolers

~~~

Feather Breathing

~~~

Feathers are a great introduction to noticing your breath. You blow, the feather moves. That is a great visual of how powerful our breath is.

Have children form a circle with their mats, and then lie on their tummies with their heads facing the center of the circle. Give everyone a feather and have them place it on the floor in front of them. When you say "GO!", everyone tries to blow their feather to the middle of the circle without moving off their mat. When all the feathers are near the middle, you can have everyone go get a new feather and repeat the activity.

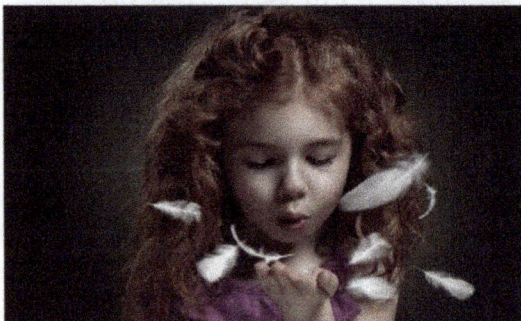

Image courtesy of Canva, Public Domain

Variations

- move mats further back each time
- have students lay on their backs and blow the feather toward the ceiling

OM tastic Yoga

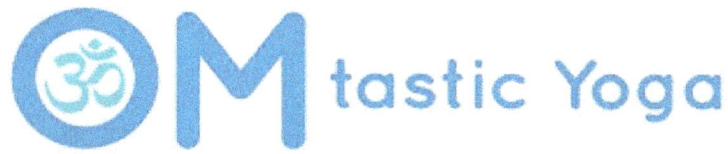

Breath Practices for Preschoolers

Hot Chocolate Breath

YOUNG STUDENTS NEED PRACTICES THAT HELP THEM CONNECT WITH THE POWER OF THEIR BREATH.

Start off by asking the children if they have ever had hot chocolate or something warm to drink on a cold day.
Ask them to tell you what this experience was like. How did it make them feel? What did they smell? What did they see?

Now, sitting on the floor or in chairs, have the students cup their hands, like they were wrapped around a mug of warm hot cocoa.
Take a slow breath in, like you are smelling the cocoa. Exhale through your mouth with pursed lips, like you are blowing to cool off the hot chocolate.
Have students practice the breath 3 more times, making the connection to breathing in that delicious smell and how the warmth travels through their body.
Ask the following questions:
What sensations do you have when you breathe in and breathe out??
Have students open their eyes and share their experiences with others.

If you can, this is a great time to have a real cup of hot chocolate

and really experience this practice.

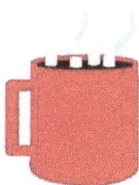

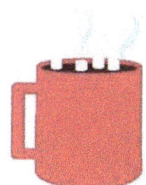

Images courtesy of Canva, Public Domain

OMtastic Yoga

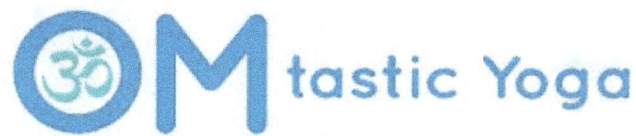

Breath Practices for Preschoolers

~~~

Ping Pong Circle Games

~~~

Have students make a circle while laying on their tummies. Have them stack their hands with elbows out to the side so that their elbows touch their neighbors. This helps to make the circle whole without any exit holes for balls.

Tell all the kids they are going to blow the balls to each other with just their breath -not hands or heads, just their breath. This is a good time to demonstrate blowing without balls and have them practice once or twice before you start.

Now, take a bag of ping pong balls, dump them in the middle, and have kids start blowing. Keep playing until it feels like it is over.

Some other ways to use ping pong balls would be to blow them with a straw, or to make a line and have students blow the balls across the room.

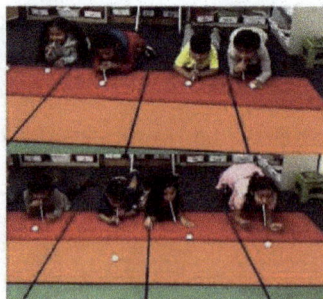

Image courtesy of Canva, Public Domain

ॐ OMtastic Yoga

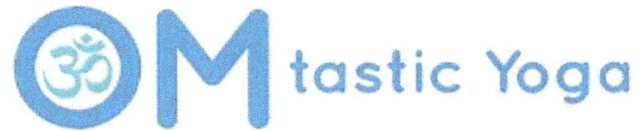

Breath Practices for Preschoolers

~~~

Pinwheel Breathing

~~~

Pinwheels can be handmade or store-bought. With this age group, if you are making pinwheels, I would do a lot of prep work ahead of time and have an extra set of hands to help put them together. Store-bought pinwheels can be bought in bulk. This is extra handy as they break often. Again, it is nice if everyone has their own.

Ways to blow:

soft
hard
slow
Run and see if the pinwheel will spin.

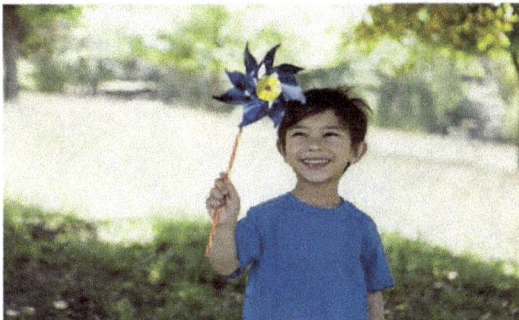

Image courtesy of Canva, Public Domain

Making a Pinwheel

Leslie Tryon
https://www.leslietryon.com/3dcolorcutout/makepinw/makeapinwheel.pdf
Instructables
https://www.instructables.com/

☉M tastic Yoga

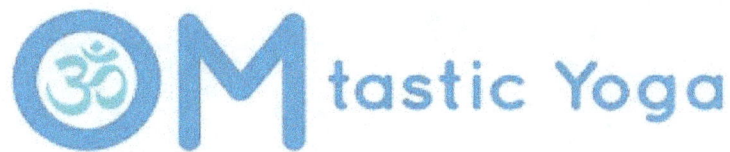

Breath Practices for Preschoolers

Pompom Breathing

Pompoms are a great tool to be able to see the power of the breath.

Pompom Breath

Have everyone line up on a starting line. Give everyone a small-sized pompom. Have them blow the pompom to the end line. Now give everyone a larger pompom. Blow it back to the first line. Which pompom was easier to blow?

You can also have kids count the number of blows it takes to go from start to finish. Can they make their blows longer so that it takes less blows to get from one side to the other?

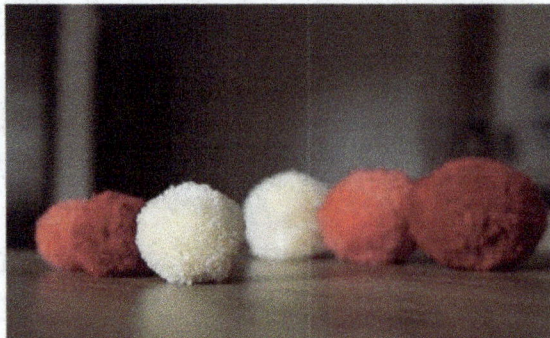

Image courtesy of Canva, Public Domain

Teacher's Notes:

_____

_____

_____

_____

_____

_____

_____

_____

_____

_____

_____

_____

_____

Teacher's Notes:

_____

_____

_____

_____

_____

_____

_____

_____

_____

_____

_____

_____

_____

_____

_____

OMtastic Yoga

CHAPTER 2

BREATH PRACTICES FOR SCHOOL AGERS

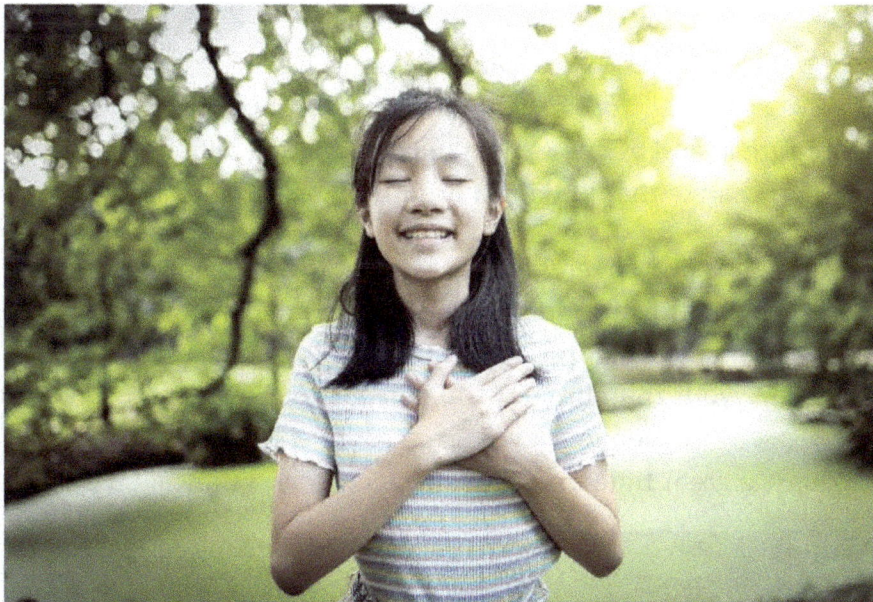

Image courtesy of Canva, Public Domain

OMtastic Yoga

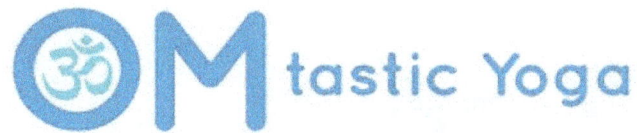

Breath Practices for School Agers

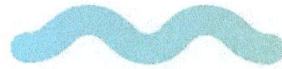

Bee Breath

Materials: none

Bee Breath can both have both an energizing and calming effect on the nervous system.

Directions

Sit tall and straight, criss-cross applesauce.
Take a deep breath in and as you exhale make a buzzing sound. Make the sound for as long as you can without taking a breath. Pause and notice how that felt.

Now take your hands and cover your ears. Take a deep breath in and buzz. Notice how this felt with your ears covered.

Lastly, gently place your thumbs over the flaps of your ears and use your fingers to cover your eyes. Buzz for one breath.
This is a great time to ask kids which version they liked best!

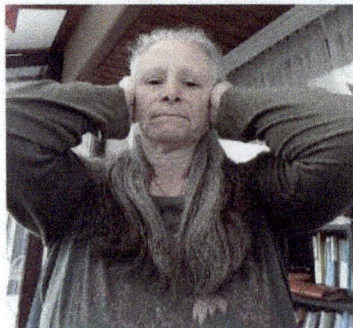

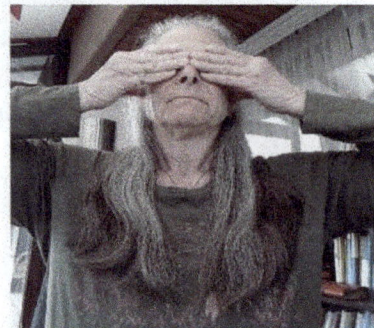

Images courtesy of Janice Pratt

OM tastic Yoga

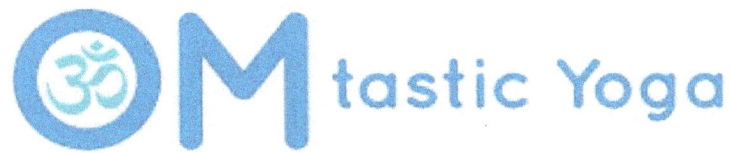

Breath Practices for School Agers

Paint a Rainbow

USE THE SONG "ALL THE COLORS OF THE RAINBOW" BY SNATAM KAUR

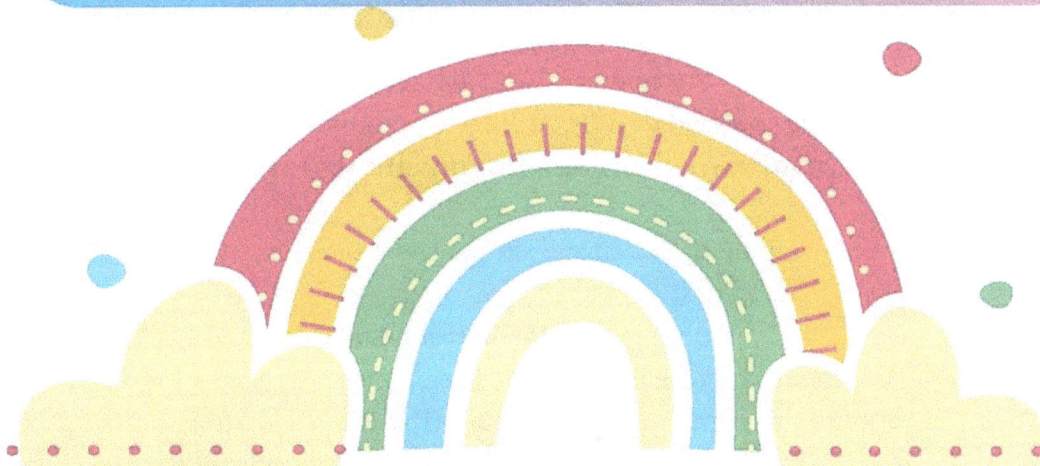

Image courtesy of Canva, Public Domain

Start the music. Standing with feet slightly apart, bring arms over to one side of your body.

As you breathe in, raise your arms over your head.

As you exhale bring them down to the other side of the body.

Reverse the movement.

To the words "Love me so" give yourself a big hug.

For eyes: Make circles like glasses and place them over over your eyes.

For smile: point to your mouth and give a big smile.

OM tastic Yoga

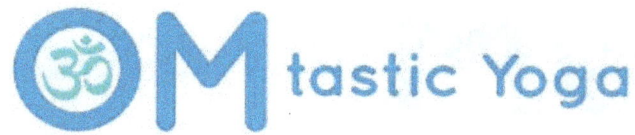

Breath Practices for School Agers

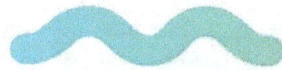

Breathing with Affirmations

Materials: none

Affirmations are very powerful and are something students can carry throughout the day. You can have students come back to their affirmation while taking a few breaths whenever needed.

Inhale the positive, exhale the negative.

Some great affirmations are:

Breathe in: I am calm.   Breathe out: Stress

Breathe in: I am strong.   Breath out: Frustration

Breathe in: I am happy.   Breathe out: Sadness

Breathe in: I love to learn.   Breathe out: Failure

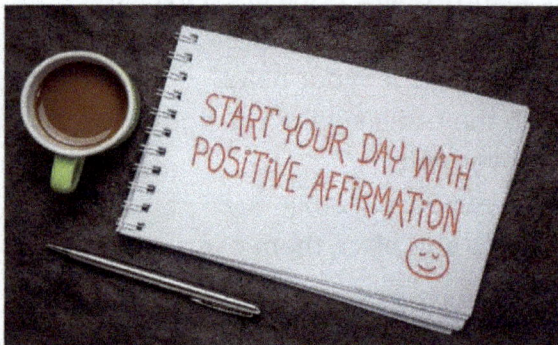

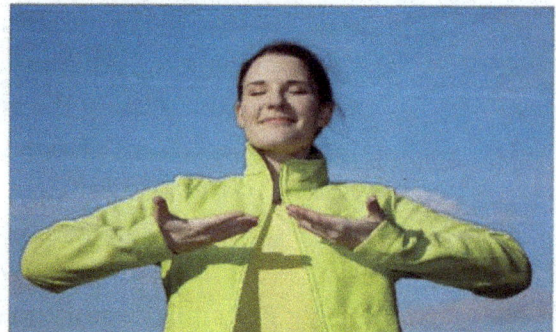

Images courtesy of Canva, Public Domain

OM tastic Yoga

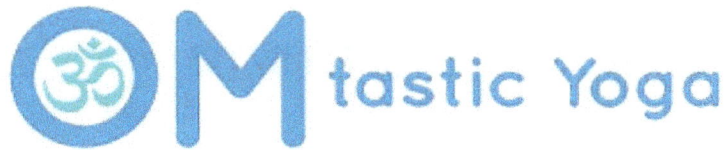

Breath Practices for School Agers

Calm Breath

Us this breath to calm the nervous system.

Sit in a comfortable position on the floor or in a chair. Make sure your back is very straight and that the top of your head is reaching toward the ceiling.

Now take a breath and think or say the following mantras:

C= Connected: I am Connected to the

Earth. A= Am: I Am me.

L= Lead: I Lead to make a difference.

M=Most: I make the Most of my life.

If you need to, you can put this mantra on an index card to help students remember it or you can make up your own mantras that go with the word: CALM Repeat several times.

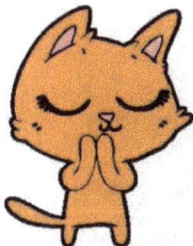

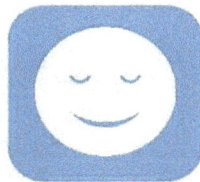

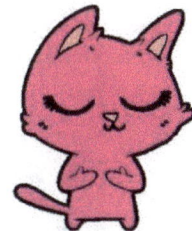

Images courtesy of Canva, Public Domain

OⓂM tastic Yoga

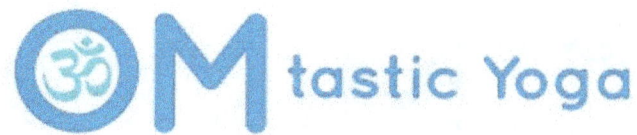

Breath Practices for School Agers

~~~

Elephant Breath

~~~

Materials: none

Elephant Breath is a breath where you sip in air and then blow it out. It is good for releasing energy and coordinating breath with movement.

Directions

Stand with your feet a little wider than hip-width apart. Bring your arms forward and interlace your fingers. Bend over with hands toward the floor, and sip in some air, like an elephant might sip in water through their trunk. As you straighten up, blow the air out, and bring the arms over the head with a slight back bend.

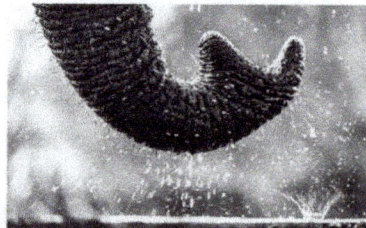

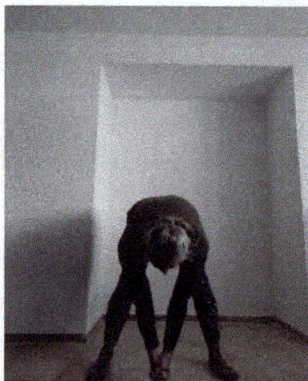

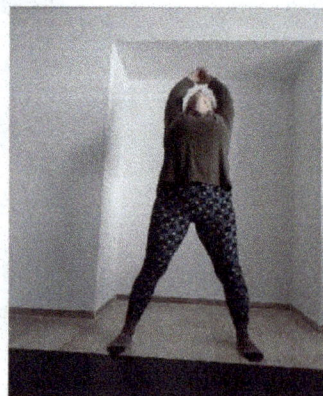

Images courtesy of Janice Pratt

OM tastic Yoga

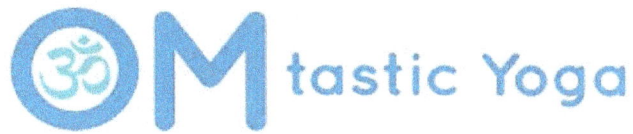

Breath Practices for School Agers

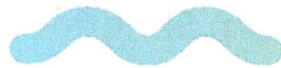

Flying Bird Breath

Materials: none

Flying Bird Breath brings movement into breath awareness. Here students work to match their breath to the movement of their arms.

Directions

Sit up tall with feet flat on the floor in a chair or seated on a cushion on the floor. Bring your arms out to the side and let your fingers rest on the floor. As you inhale, bring your arms over your head, trying to end the inhale as your fingers touch. Exhale as you lower you arms, trying to make sure that your fingers touch the floor as you finish the exhale. Repeat for several more smooth, slow breaths.

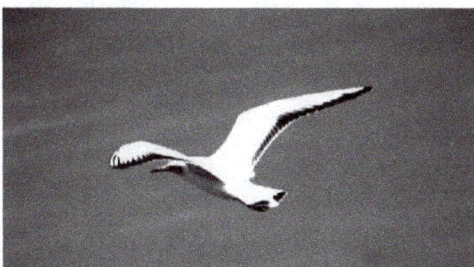

Inhale, arms move up.

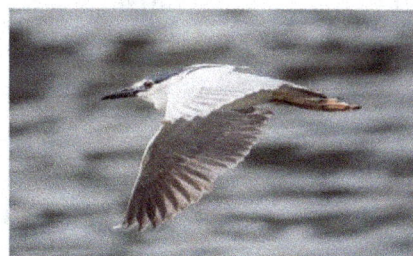

Exhale, arms move down.

Images courtesy of Canva, Public Domain

OMtastic Yoga

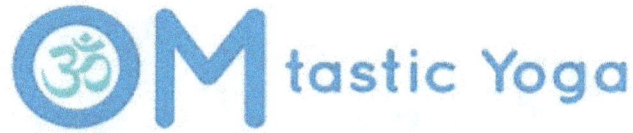

Breath Practices for School Agers

Hoberman Sphere Breath

Materials: Hoberman Sphere

A Hoberman's sphere is a great tool for being able to control the rate of the breath.

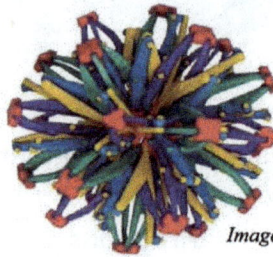

Image cortesy of Canva, Public Domain

It is great if everyone can have their own sphere to practice with, but you can also take turns. It is also great to have those who are waiting for their turn to touch all their fingers together, and then expand their fingers as they breath in. When they exhale, they bring their fingers back together. They are mimicking the motion of the sphere.

With the sphere, as you inhale expand the ball matching the rate of the expansion of the ball to the rate of your in breath. As you exhale, slowly bring the ball back to the orginial shape. Here, students are matching their breath to the visual movement of the ball.

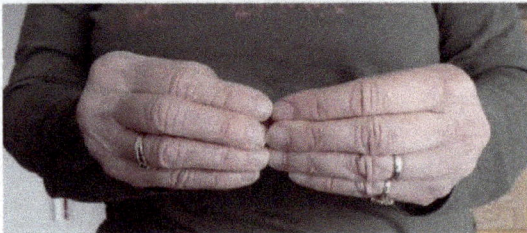

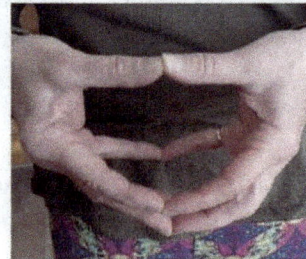

Images courtesy of Janice Pratt

ॐ**OM** tastic Yoga

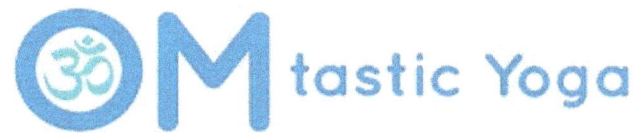

Breath Practices for School Agers

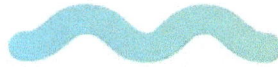

〜

Ocean Breath

〜

Materials: none

Ocean Breath is a warming and energizing breath.

Directions
With students sitting up tall, have
students hold up their hand in front of their mouth. Tell them to pretend it is
a mirror. Take a breath in, and make the "ha" sound, like you are
trying to fog up a mirror. Practice this a couple of times. Now, have students
close their lips, take a deep breath in and, as they exhale make the
"ha" sound at the back of their throat. It might sound like the
ocean or a "Darth Vader" sound. Try it a few more
times. As students get better at this breath, they can do the breath as they are
doing yoga poses. Students can also work on making the breath steady and smooth.

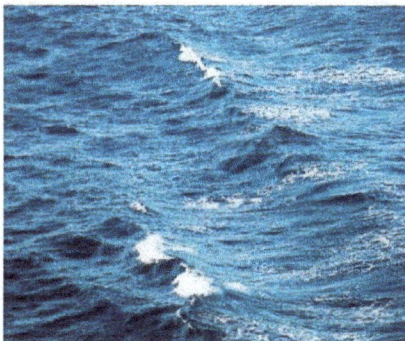

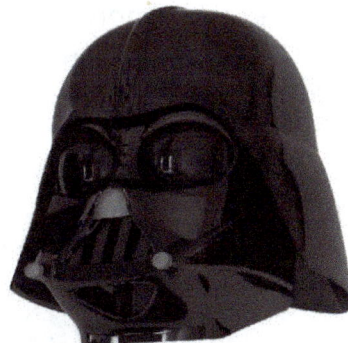

Images courtesy of Canva, Public Domain

OM tastic Yoga

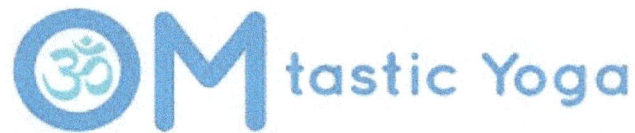

Breath Practices for School Agers

STAIR STEP BREATH

Materials: none

Stair-step breathing is good for the release of fear, anxiety, and stress.

Directions

Have students sit up nice and tall, either sitting on the floor or
in a chair. If in a chair, make sure that their feet are flat on the floor and
they are sitting up tall, away from the back of the chair.
Explain that everyone is going to take in 3 sips of air as if they are climbing up the
ladder on a sliding board.
When they get their lungs full of air, they exhale
through the mouth, imagining that the breath is smooth, just like sliding down
the slide. Repeat a few times. When students feel comfortable with the
routine, you can ask them to sip in 3 sips of air and pause at the top,
look out, and imagine something beautiful, then let their breath slide
out. When students are more comfortable with this breath, they might find that they
can take in 4 or 5 sips of air to fill their lungs.

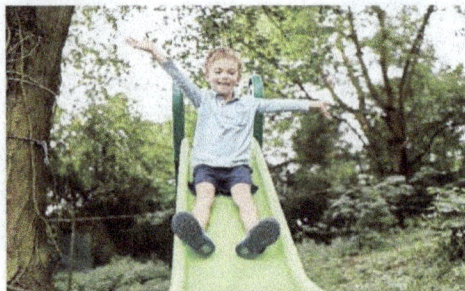

Image courtesy of Canva, Public Domain

Teacher's Notes:

_____

_____

_____

_____

_____

_____

_____

_____

_____

_____

_____

_____

_____

_____

Teacher's Notes:

_____

_____

_____

_____

_____

_____

_____

_____

_____

_____

_____

_____

_____

OM tastic Yoga

CHAPTER 3

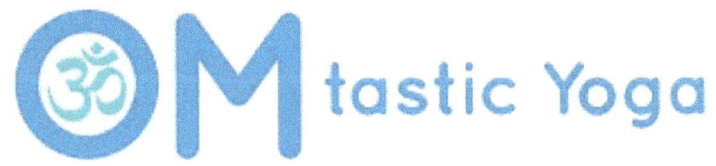

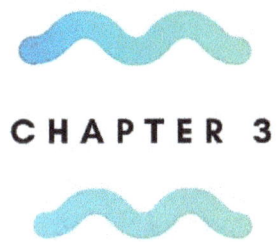

BREATH PRACTICES FOR THE CLASSROOM

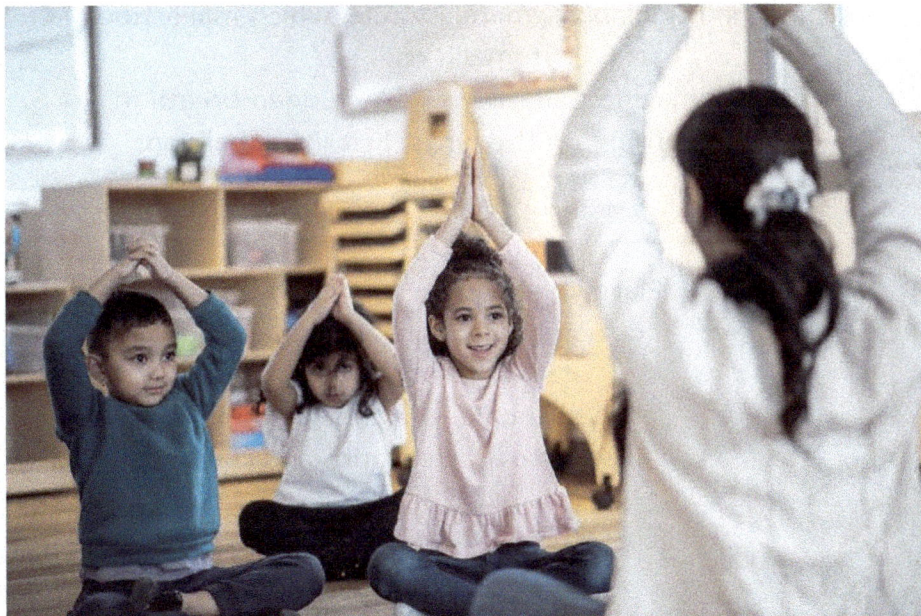

Image courtesy of Canva, Public Domain

OMtastic Yoga

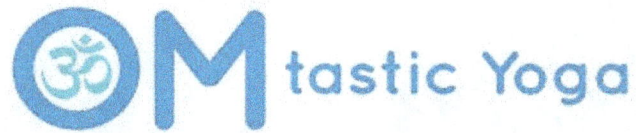

Breath Practices for the Classroom

Balloon Breathing

Balloon breathing is all about learning to bring the air all the way down into the lower lungs. The science behind this breath is that when the lungs fill, they push on the diaphragmatic muscle, which makes the stomach rise.
You can imagine that, as you take a deep breath in, the air is filling up the lungs, just like a balloon.

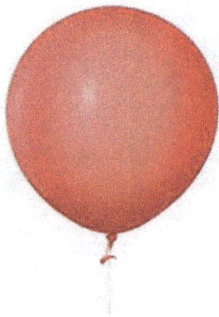

Place one hand on your stomach and one hand on your heart. Either sit up tall, or lie on your back.
As you inhale, imagine your lungs filling with air. Belly, ribs and chest.

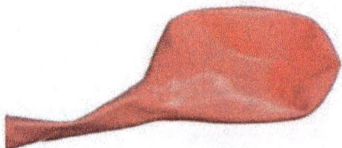

As you exhale, imagine the air leaving the balloon. Let your belly fall toward your spine.

Support Materials for Balloon Breathing

There are some great crafts that you can do with this breath. Here are a few links for you to explore.

Model of a Lung: https://www.youtube.com/watch?v=CBv2BqqAydE
How to Make a Model of a Lung: https://www.instructables.com/Make-a-Human-Lung-Model/
Building a Lung Model :(https://ctsciencecenter.org/blog/science-at-play-make-your-own-lung-model/#:~:text=Tape%20two%20balloons%20on%20the,to%20see%20both%20lungs%20inflate!

And some great videos:

Two-minute mindfulness: Ballon Breathing: https://www.youtube.com/watch?v=2PcCmxEW5WA

How to Practice Balloon Breathing:https://www.youtube.com/watch?v=GLjSXJBHszM

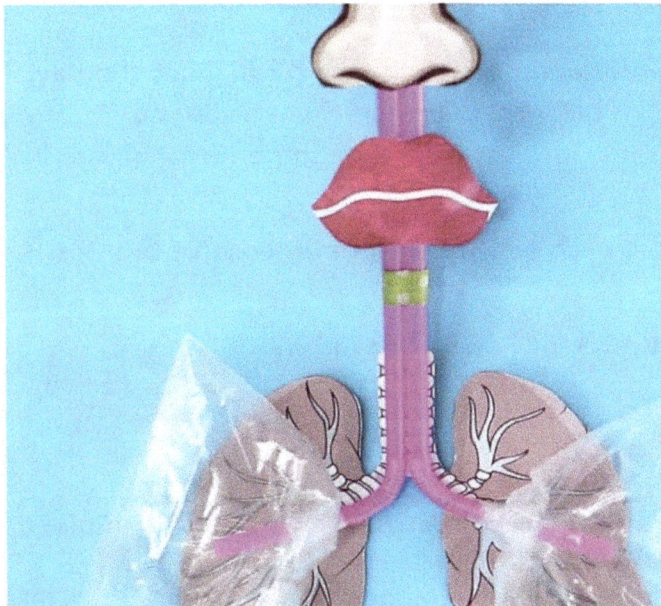

Audio recording of belly breath meditation
https://www.dropbox.com/
s/4zen200nariqxeo/balloon%20belly%20%281%29.wav?dl=0

OMtastic Yoga

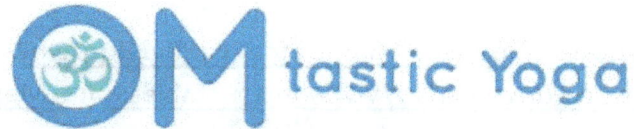

Breath Practice for the Classroom

Breathing in the Good, Breathing out the Bad

Listen to the recording, either with your class or as a
tool for you to be able to lead
this activity yourself.

The affirmations can change throughout the day,
tailoring them to fit whatever you
are getting ready to do next.

Start each activity with three positive breaths.

Breathe in "Peace." Breathe out "Anger."

Video for "Breathing Good In, Breathing Bad Out"
https://www.dropbox.com/scl/fi/b9c4bt1xvbv1qav6bfe5d/Good-
In_Bad-Out-Breath-Exercise-by-Cole-Harding.m4a?
rlkey=j5jubml39v1b65nop1ejqdem7&dl=0

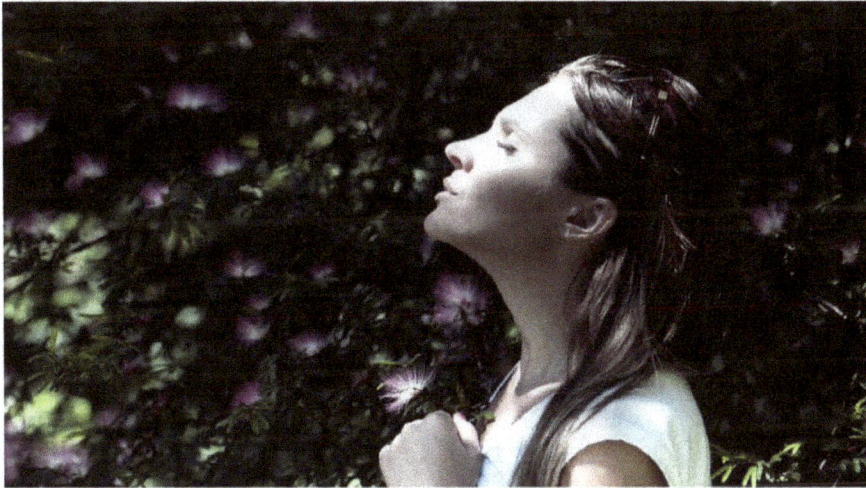

Image courtesy of Canva, Public Domain

Script for Breathing in the Good, Breathing Out the Bad

This breathing exercise is a calming breath to help us stay
positive as negative thoughts come up during our class and learning.
We will do this breath together to try and get a head start
focusing on the positive.
Sit up tall and shut your eyes.
Think of a positive thought such as " I can do my best."

Repeat: "I can do my best" to yourself.

Take a deep breath in, for the count of five.

Breathe in this positive thought and let it fill your whole being.

Breathe out slowly, letting go of all the negative thoughts or energy that
comes up.

Breathe in, "I can do my best".

Imagine the positive thought coming into your body and
filling you up from top to bottom, your whole being.

Imagine breathing out all of the negative energy, letting it
slide away out the door, away from this room.

Let's do this for 3 more breaths.
Let your breath come back to normal for a couple more breaths, soaking in
that positive focus, as we prepare to learn.

OMtastic Yoga

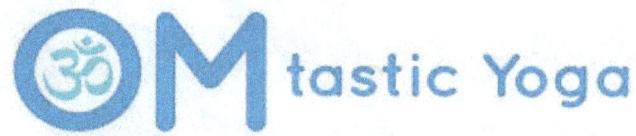

Breath Practices for the Classroom

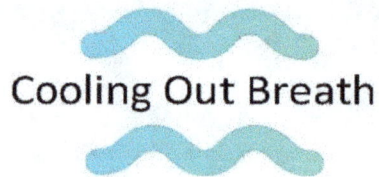

Cooling Out Breath

This activity can be done with students in a classroom when you notice a particularly high level of energy in your group, or when there is a great deal of conflict.

Some great times might be:

- after recess
- after PE
- after students have gone through a transition
- at the beginning of and after school yoga class
- after a high energy class

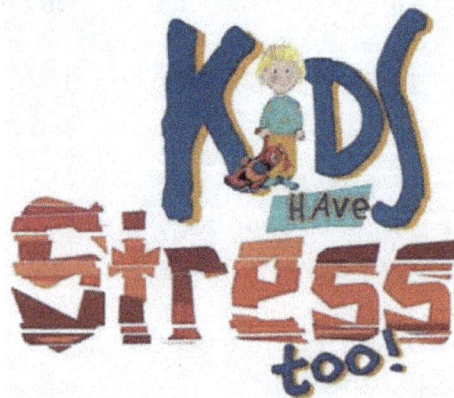

Image courtesy of Canva, Public Domain

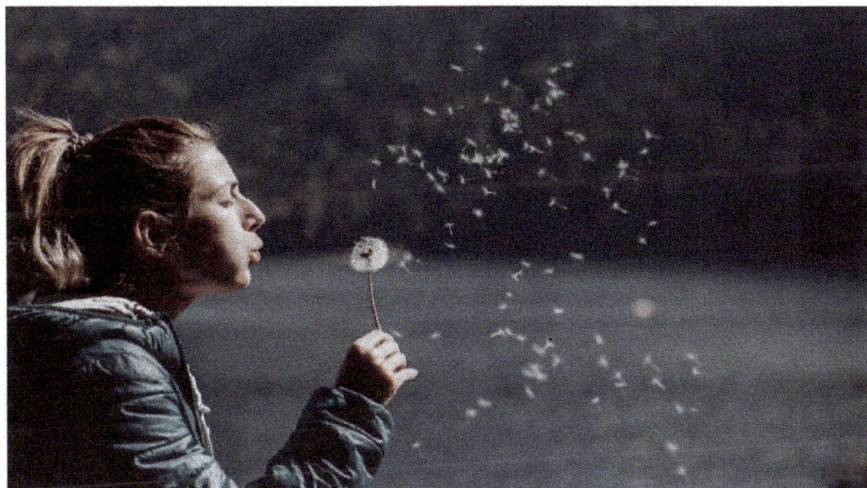

Image courtesy of Canva, Public Domain

Script for Cooling Out Breath

Have students sit in a circle on a rug. If space is limited, they can stand in a circle.

Turn off or dim overhead lights if possible.

You could start by describing what you are noticing in student voices, their body language, their level of activity. Let them know they are going to practice a way to use their breath to help manage their energy, so that they can work on an activity that requires focus and concentration.

Ask everyone to take a breath in with you, and blow it out very slowly through pursed lips, like you are blowing softly on a candle. Repeat several times until you notice the energy of the group changing.

You can also have children say **"aaaahhhhh"** softly as they exhale. To make it fun you can start with a louder "aaahhh" or change the intonation of the "aaahhh." Make the sound go up and down.

End the activity with the soft, slow out-breath without sound, for the last couple of breaths.

OM tastic Yoga

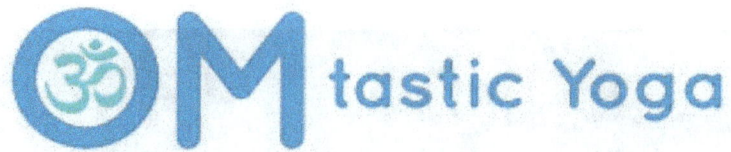

Breath Practices for the Classroom

Color Breathing

HAVE A DISCUSSION ABOUT HOW COLORS CAN MAKE US FEEL DIFFERENT WAYS.

Have students sit up straight and tall.
If it is okay, they can close their eyes or, with younger kids you can
hold up different colored paper.
Now breathe in (red, or blue...). Notice what thoughts come up as you
breathe and think of this color.
There is no right or wrong, just notice.
Now breathe out the same color.
Continue with a few different colors.
After breathing in colors, take a deep breath in and imagine that you are
breathing in all the colors of the rainbow.
How does this make you feel?

Let kids share their experience.

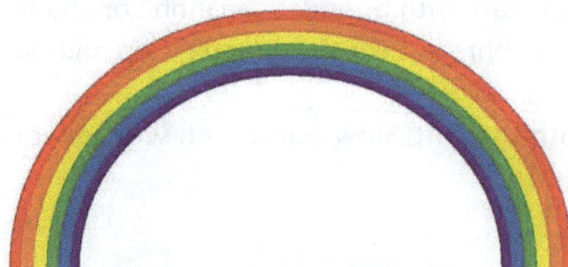

Image courtesy of Canva, Public Domain

OMtastic Yoga

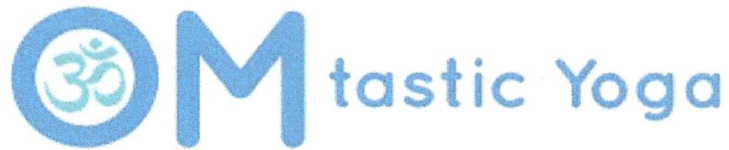

Breath Practice for the Classroom

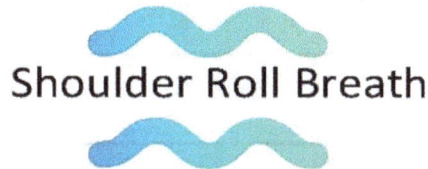

Shoulder Roll Breath

CONNECT BREATH WITH MOVEMENT TO RELEASE NECK TENSION

This exercise will help children connect with their bodies through a breathing activity. We often carry a lot of stress in our neck which demonstrates one way our bodies react to stress. This is a simple activity to support the body.

Children can close their eyes or have a softened gaze while completing this exercise. It is important to do what is comfortable. Children can be seated in a circle, facing the center as they do this guided exercise together or, if children feel self-conscious, everyone can face the outside of the circle. Students will be asked to complete 5-6 breaths and then provide feedback on their experience.

First, have children raise their shoulder toward their ears and then let them drop. Repeat several times. Now, as you raise the shoulders, breathe in. As you exhale, let the shoulder drop. This may be enough for younger kids.

The next option would be to roll the shoulders up and back on the inhale. On the exhale, the shoulders move toward the front of the body. Repeat for several rounds. Then, reverse the direction of the roll.

Teacher's Notes:

_____

_____

_____

_____

_____

_____

_____

_____

_____

_____

_____

_____

_____

Teacher's Notes:

_____

_____

_____

_____

_____

_____

_____

_____

_____

_____

_____

_____

_____

OMtastic Yoga

CHAPTER 4

BREATH PRACTICES FOR TEEN/TWEENS

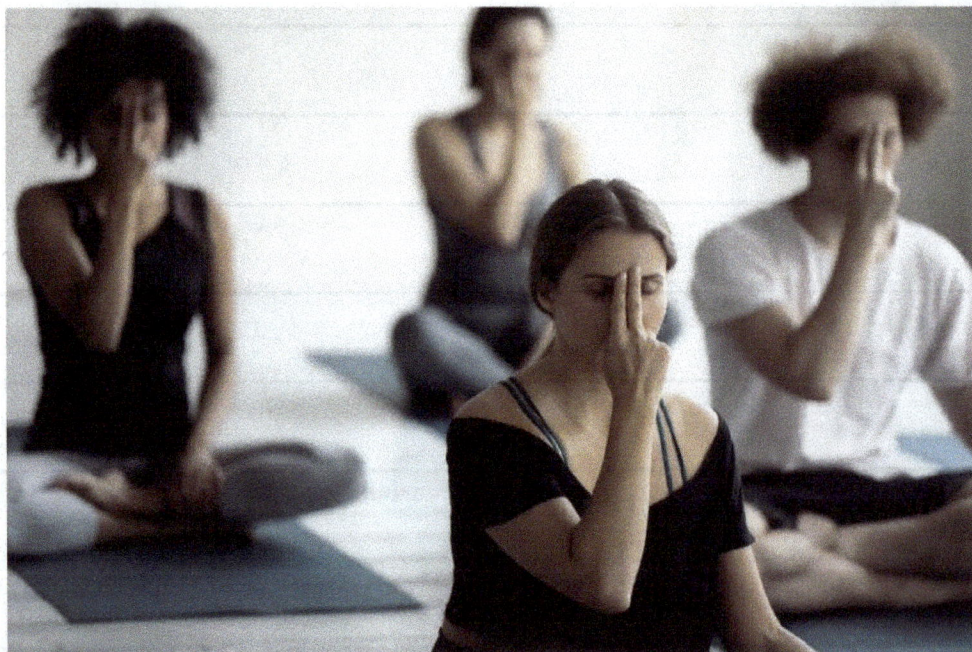

Image courtesy of Canva, Public Domain

OM tastic Yoga

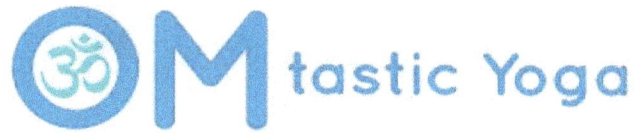

Breath Practices for Teens/Tweens

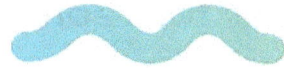

Alternate Nostril Breath

Materials: none

Alternate nostril breath is a breath that balances both sides of the brain. It can have a very calming effect on the nervous system and is great for anxiety and depression.

Directions

Sit up tall with feet flat on the floor in a chair or seated on a cushion. During the breath, you will place your thumb lightly on your right nostril with your ring finger gently on your left nostril. The thumb and ring finger will gently close off the respective sides of the nostrils as you breathe through the opposite side.

Begin by gently closing the right nostril. Inhale through the left. Gently close of the left nostril and exhale through the right. Now, inhale through the right, close off the right nostril and exhale through the left. Inhale through the left. Close off the left nostril and exhale right.

Continue for several rounds.

Finish with an exhale on the left side.

Drop your hands and notice the effect on the mind, the body, and the spirit.

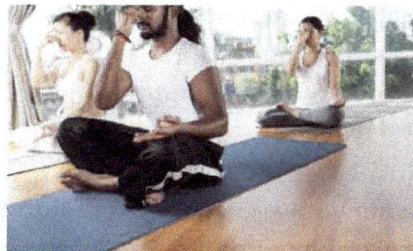

The two middle fingers can rest on the forehead or can curl in and rest on the palm.

Image courtesy of Canva, Public Domain

43

OMtastic Yoga

Breath Practices for Teens and Tweens

Back-to-Back Breathing

Materials: a partner

Back-to-Back breathing allows students to tune into their partners breath. This can take some concentration and focus. One benefit is that of connection. We know that simple touch can release hormones that make us feel good. This can really lift moods and produce a sense of calm.

Directions

Have students sit criss-cross applesauce with backs touching. It is helpful if students are close in height so that their backs match in size. However, this is not a deal breaker if there is a size difference.
The kids are touching backs but not pushing on each other. Just firm pressure, so that they can feel their partners back all along the spine.

Go ahead and close the eyes, or look softly at the ground. Bring your attention to the breath.
As you feel your breath become steady, bring your attention to the back of your body and see if you can feel the inhales and exhales of your partner. Both partners may need to take deeper breaths with long, slow inhales and long, slow exhales to make the breath "feel-able".
When you have a good feeling of your partner's breath, see if you can begin to match your breath to your partner's breath. Take 3 more breaths together.
Now let your breath return to normal.
Turn around and thank your partner.

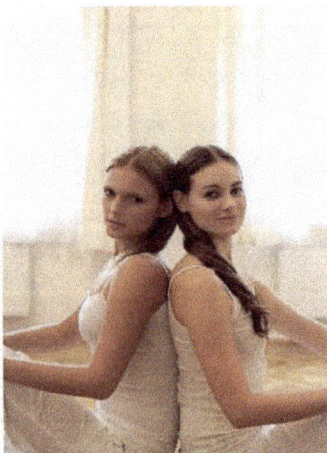

Image courtesy of Canva, Public Domain

ॐOM tastic Yoga

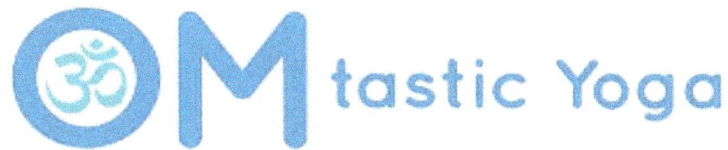

Breath Practices for Teens/Tweens

Drawing Your Breath

Material: paper and a dark marker

This activity is so simple but always seems to amaze kids. "Drawing Your Breath" is an across age level activity, but can really move to a deep level in teens and tweens.

Directions

Find a comfortable seat and place your paper in front of you.

Now, place you marker on one spot on the paper.

In a moment, everyone will close their eyes or look away from their papers.

They will start to notice their breath.

Move you maker for each inhale and each exhale.

Continue breathing and drawing until I say to stop.

Begin.

Remember to move your marker in a different direction each time you inhale and each time you exhale.

Stop.

Open your eyes and look at your drawing of your breath.

(You can choose to have everyone show their drawings, commenting on the fact that each of us is different and so is our breath pattern.)

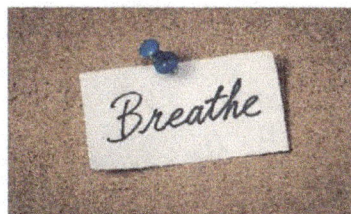

Image courtesy of Canva, Public Domain

OMtastic Yoga

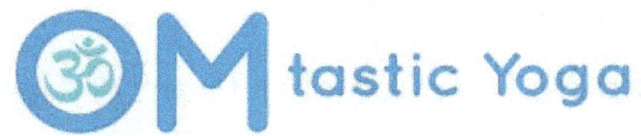

Breath Practices for Teens and Tweens

Horse Lips Breath

Horse Lips Breath is a great way to wake up and lighten the mood in a group. It is fun to flutter the lips and release energy.

Have students sit up tall.
Notice the breath as it is.

Now take a deep breath in. Exhale and flutter the breath through the lips.

Notice the vibration on the lips and enjoy the sound of the breath. Repeat several times.

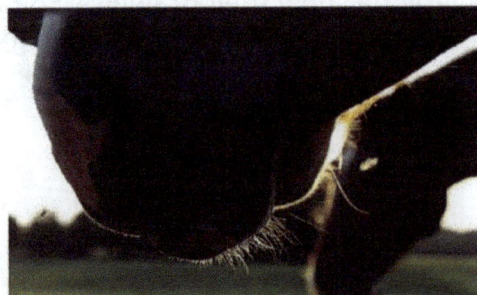

Image courtesy of Canva, Public Domain

OMtastic Yoga

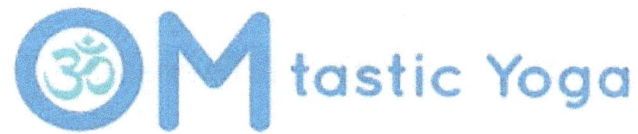

Breath Practices for Teens and Tweens

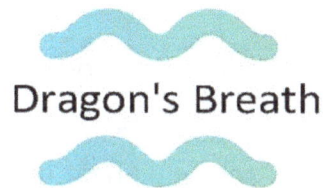

Dragon's Breath

Dragon's breath is a great way to let off steam.

Sit on your knees with your seat on your heals.
Take a deep breath in and as you exhale, stick out your tongue, and make the "haaaa" sound.
Repeat this breath three times while thinking of something you need to let go of!

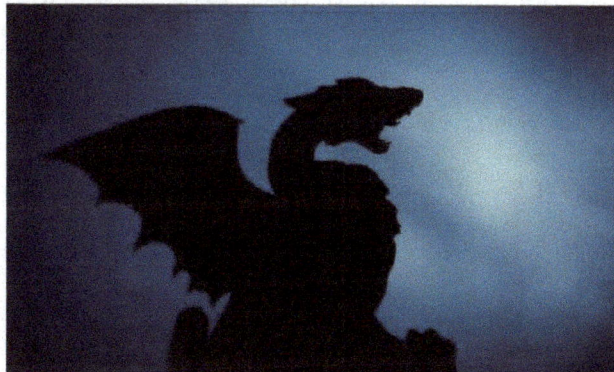

Image courtesy of Canva, Public Domain

ॐ OM tastic Yoga

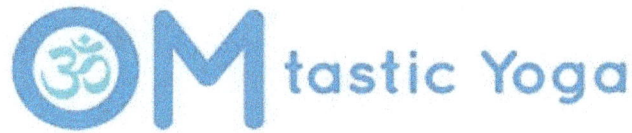

Breath Practices for Teens and Tweens

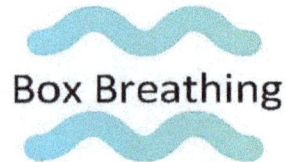

Box Breathing

Materials: none

Box breathing can be done while tracing a finger on a surface, in the air, or with just the visualization of the shape of a square. This breath has a slight hold as you move across the top and bottom of the square, but should not feel constricting in any way. Students can move at their own pace to make it a smooth breath. This breath is good for calming the nervous system and can feel very grounding.

Directions

Sit up tall with feet flat on the floor, in a chair or seated on a cushion on the floor. Think of the shape of a square as you inhale. Imagine your breath moving up the left side of the square. At the top of the inhale, suspend your breath as you imagine moving across the top of the square. Exhale as you imagine the right side of the square. Suspend your breath as you move across the bottom of the square. Repeat for several complete rounds of breath.
Notice the effect on the mind, the body, and the spirit.

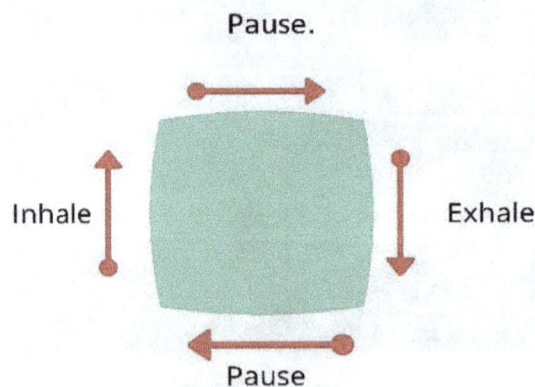

Pause.

Inhale   Exhale

Pause

Image courtesy of Canva, Public Domain

OMtastic Yoga

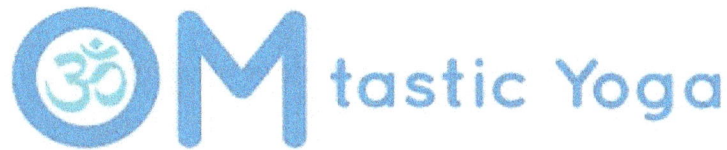

Breath Practices for Teens and Tweens

Staircase Breathing

Materials: none

Staircase breath is a fun activity for older kids. However, you must consider how familiar the students are with each other, because students will be putting their head on their neighbor's belly. You might use caution at certain ages when doing this in mixed gender groups. Because you will be making a chain of students laying down, it also takes a bit of room to do this activity.

Directions

Have one student lie down on their back off to one side of the space you have. Have them put their arm out that is on the side toward where there is the most space in the room. (See the picture below.)

The next person will put their head on the belly of the first person, and then put out their arm that will be close to the body of the first person.

Keep repeating until all students are lying in this manner.

The first goal will to be to pass the sound "ha" down the line. The first person will make a loud "ha" sound. When the second person feels and hears the sound, then they will also make the sound. Pass this sound in this way, all the way down the line. At this point, kids might start giggling or laughing and, of course, that is part of the fun of this activity.

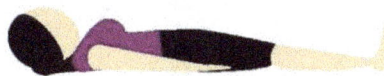

Image courtesy of Canva, Public Domain

"Staircase Breathing" continued

After this you can send a chains of "ha's" down the row. You can do two "ha's"
then 3 and more until everyone is laughing!

After the laughter dies down, ask everyone to just settle in, close their eyes, and
see if they can feel the fall and rise of the belly on which their
head is resting.
Notice how that breath feels on their head and neck.
Notice how it feels to be this close to friends.
No emotion is right or wrong. Just take time to notice.
Now see if you can match your breath to the breath of your neighbor.
If each person in the line works to breath with the person they are
resting on, soon all of you will be breathing as one.
Notice how this feels.
Take one more deep breath together, and then come back to
your own breath.
Blink your eyes open and slowly sit up.
Thank your partners with some kind of sign-a bow of the head, namaste hands,
a high five or even a hug.

As a group, you can discuss the effects of this breath activity.

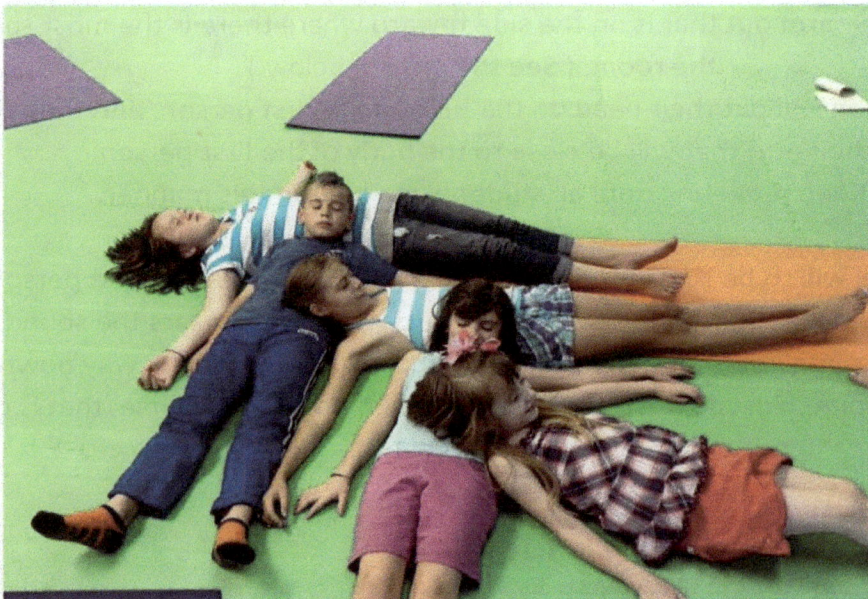

Image courtesy of Canva, Public Domain

Teacher's Notes:

_____

_____

_____

_____

_____

_____

_____

_____

_____

_____

_____

_____

_____

Teacher's Notes:

_____

_____

_____

_____

_____

_____

_____

_____

_____

_____

_____

_____

_____

OMtastic Yoga

CHAPTER 5

BREATH PRACTICES FOR ALL AGES

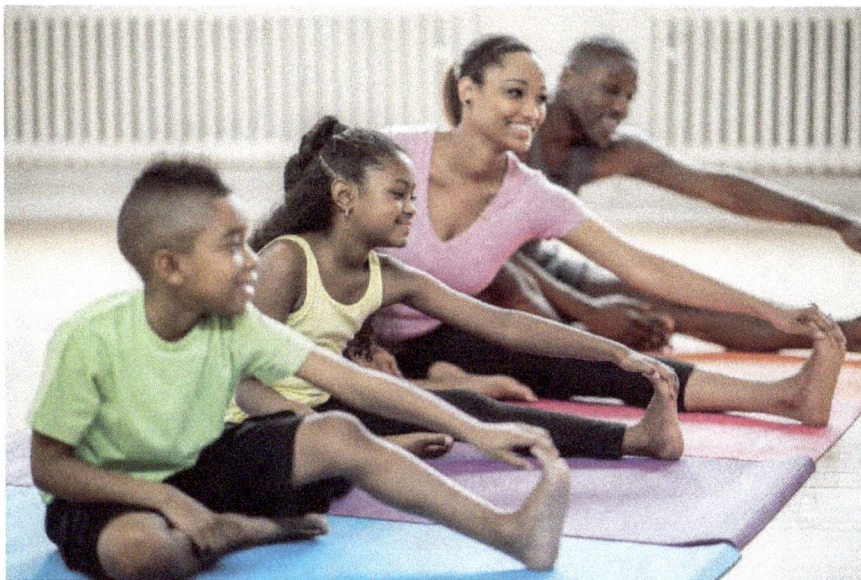

Image courtesy of Canva, Public Domain

ॐ OM tastic Yoga

Breath Practices for All Ages

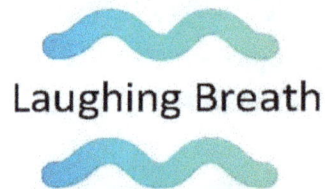

Laughing Breath

Materials: none

As a group, take a collective breath with a log slow exhale. Have
everyone think of something that was funny to them. Now, on the count of 3,
everyone starts laughing. It might be a fake laugh at first,
but as everyone starts laughing, it usually catches on. Laugh until
everyone naturally stops.
Notice how it feels to let go and really laugh!

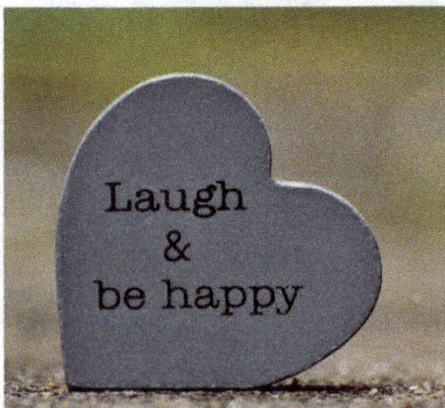

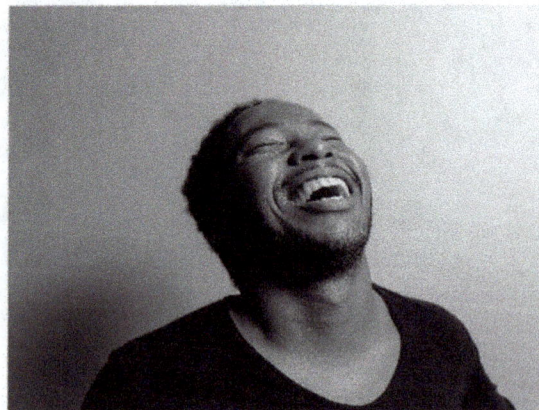

Images courtesy of Canva, Public Domain

OMtastic Yoga

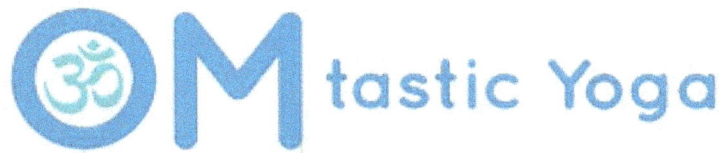

Breath Practices for All Ages

Shape Breathing

BREATHING WITH A SHAPE CAN HELP REMIND US TO TAKE CONTROLLED BREATHS AND TO PACE OUR BREATHING.

Circle Breath
Using the pattern or drawing the shape in the air, start at the top of the circle, and inhale as you move your finger to the bottom. Pause at the bottom, and then exhale as you move your finger toward the top of the circle.
Repeat.

Box Breathing
Using the pattern or drawing the shape in the air, start at one corner of the square-inhale as you move your finger across the side and pause as your finger moves along the next side. Then exhale as you move your finger along the third side, and then pause the breath on the fourth side.
Repeat.

Figure 8 Breathing
Start in the middle of the shape. Inhale on one loop of the figure-8, back to the middle and then exhale on the other side of the loop.
Repeat.

Triangle Breathing
Starting at the top of the triangle, inhale along one side, pause at the bottom side, and then exhale toward the top of the triangle.
Repeat.

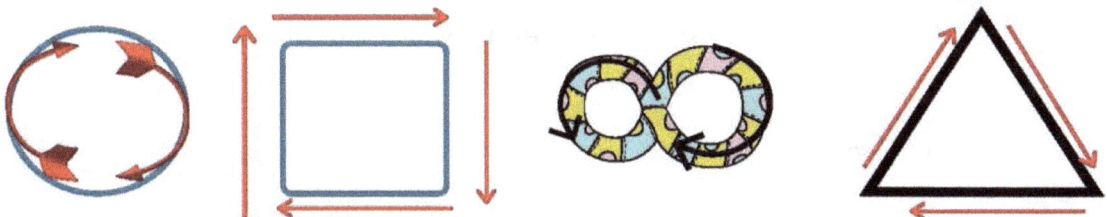

Images courtesy of Canva, Public Domain

OM tastic Yoga

Breath Practices for All Ages

Breath Rhymes

RHYMES CAN HELP YOU TO REMEMBER AN ORDER OR A SKILL. TRY THESE RHYMES TO HELP YOU REMEMBER TO BREATHE SLOWLY.

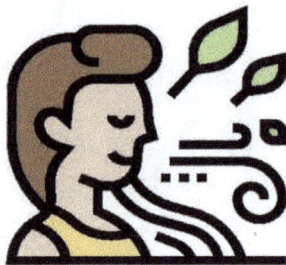

Rhyme 1

Breathe in long
Blow out slow
Now I know
I am ready to go!

Rhyme 2
I breathe in- I am still
I breath out- I let go
I breathe in- I feel quiet
I breathe out- I am at peace.

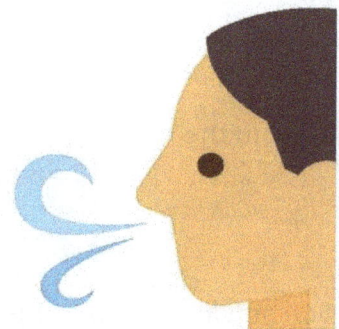

Rhyme 3

Fill my lungs,
Then empty them out.
That is what breathing is all about!

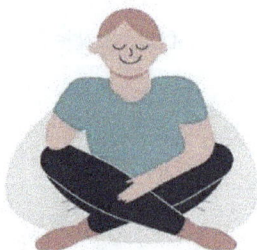

Images courtesy of Canva, Public Domain

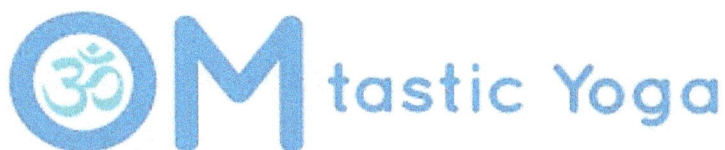

OMtastic Yoga

Breath Practices for All Ages

Reach and Breathe

STRETCHING THE ARMS IN DIFFERENT WAYS CAN HELP TO OPEN THE RIBCAGE AND MAKE MORE ROOM FOR THE BREATH.

Version 1
Start with your fingers touching your shoulders. As you inhale lift both arms toward the sky.
As you exhale, lower your arms back to your shoulder.
Repeat several times.

With this breath you can do one arm at a time or reach to opposite corners of the room across the body.

Version 2
Take a breath in.
As you interlace your fingers, flip your palms away from your chest on the exhale.
Inhale-arms to the sky with fingers still interlaced, palms facing the sky.
Exhale-arms to chest, palms toward the chest.
Repeat.

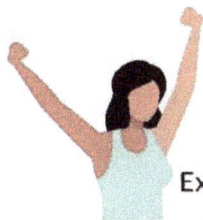

Version 3
Namaste hands in front of the chest. Inhale.
Exhale- round back and push arms forward. Inhale-open arms wide and lift chest toward the sky. Exhale arms to chest in Namaste.

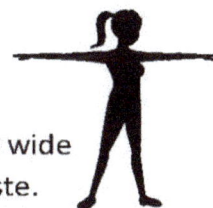

Images courtesy of Canva, Public Domain

OMtastic Yoga

Breath Practice for All Ages

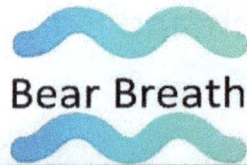

Bear Breath

LET'S PRETEND THAT YOU ARE A BEAR. THIS BREATH WILL HAVE YOU MAKING A LOW GROWLING NOISE IN YOUR THROAT.

Sit up or stand tall.
Take a breath in.
As you exhale, make a low growling sound in the back of your throat.
It may be a bit hard to make this sound low and soft. You might need to practice a few times.
You might think of gargling with the growl sound!

Try this a few times.
How did this breath make you feel?

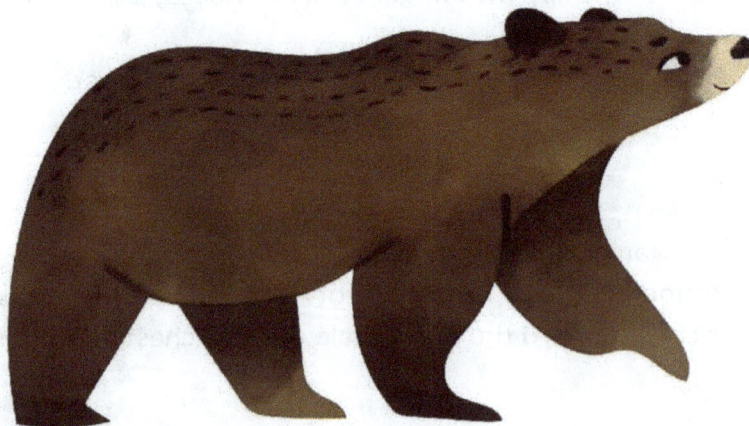

Image courtesy of Canva, Public Domain

OM tastic Yoga

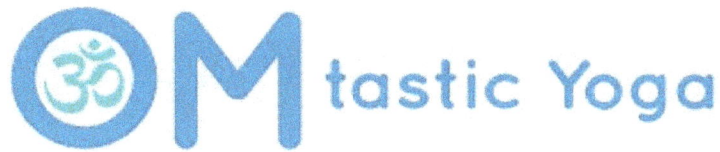

Breath Practice for All Ages

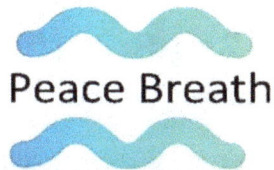

Peace Breath

HOW DO WE FEEL PEACE IN OUR MINDS AND BODIES? SOMETIMES IT TAKES A QUIET MOMENT TO FIND THIS PEACE.

Sit up or stand tall.
Take a deep breath in. As you exhale, softly say the word "Peace."

Notice how you feel when you say this word.
What do you picture in your mind when you say "Peace"?
Repeat several times.
You may close your eyes if you like and picture a
place that feels peaceful.
How does your body feel when you think about
something peaceful?
Can you think of a time this breath might be useful?

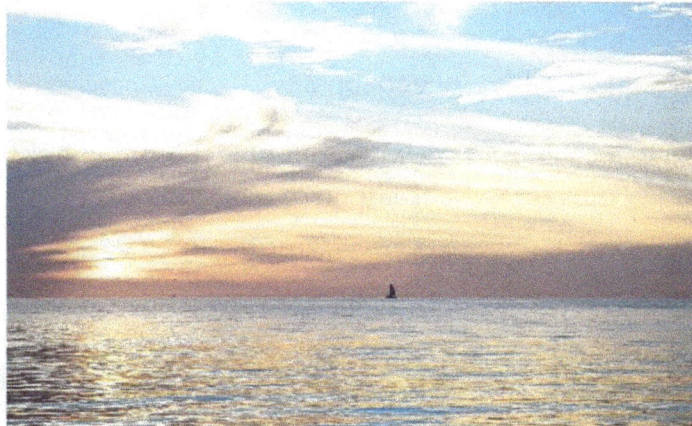

Image courtesy of Canva, Public Domain

OMtastic Yoga

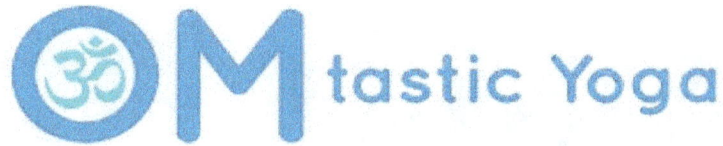

Breath Practices for All Ages

Bean Bag Breathing

Coordinating breath with movement can really help the brain and body connect. Use a bean bag, a small ball, a small stuffie, or other small item you can hold easily in one hand.

Version 1

Sit in a comfortable position on the floor or in a chair. Stretch your arms out to the side. Hold your object in one hand. As you breathe in, lift your arms up over your head and transfer the item from one hand to the other. As you exhale, bring the arms out parallel to the floor. Repeat several times.

Version 2

Sit in a comfortable position on the floor or in a chair.
Stretch your arms out to the side. Hold your object in one hand. As you breath in, lift your arms up over your head and transfer the item from one hand to the other. As you exhale, bring the arms down to the floor, switching the item from hand to hand behind your back. Repeat several times.

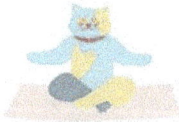

Version 3

Make up your own breath pattern with your object. Remember to make each movement a breath in or a breath out.

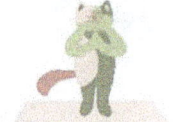

Find your SUPERPOWER!

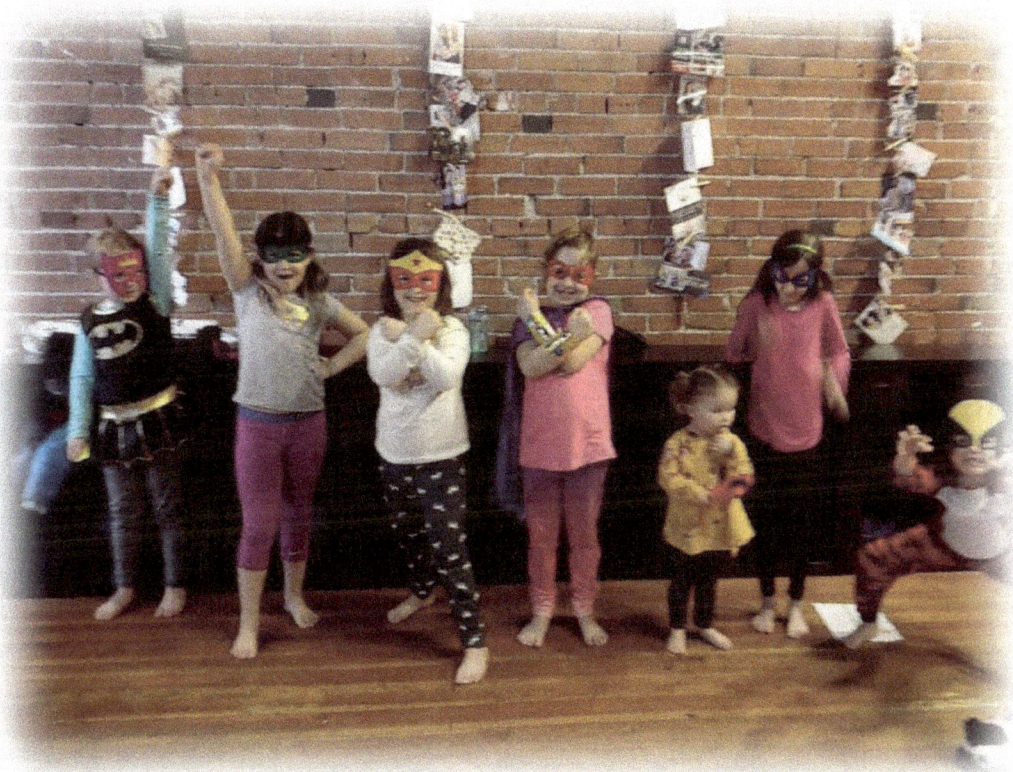

Image courtesy of Janice Pratt

BREATHE!

Acknowledgments

I am thankful for all the students who have learned with me over the years, all the parents who have entrusted their children to the practices of yoga, and the many mentors who have taught me the yoga path.

Namaste

About the Author

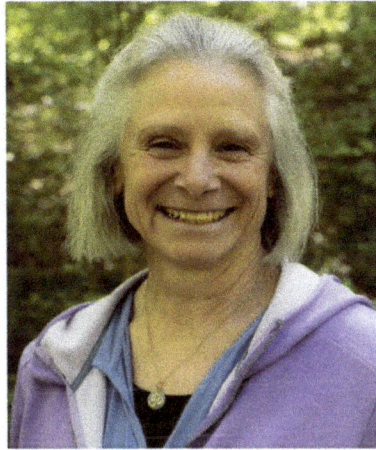

Image courtesy of Janice Pratt

Janice Pratt has been a "yogi in training" for the past 25 years. Jan found that yoga was a great complement to gymnastics, dance, and hiking and that a yoga mat could travel anywhere! She has been fortunate enough to train at yoga ashrams in both Austria and Germany. She is 200 RYA trained, trained in Accessible Yoga and Karma Kids yoga.

Janice has also been passionate about children for most of her life. While having 4 children of her own, she has also owned a preschool, been a children's librarian, and worked in public schools.

Janice currently is busy writing a series of books designed to empower children to pursue their dreams. For more information on her books go to: www.janpratt.com

"Children are natural yogis,ready to explore their world with their mind, body, and spirit. Join us and play!"

www.omtastic-yoga.com